Learn and Live

Family & Friends®
CPR
STUDENT MANUAL

Editors

Louis Gonzales, BS, LP,
Senior Science Editor
Michael W. Lynch, NREMT-P,
Content Consultant

Senior Managing Editor

Sue Bork

Special Contributors

Richard DeLisi, NREMT-B
Susan Fuchs, MD
Barbara Furry, RNC, MS, CCRN
Mary Mast, RN
Mark A. Terry, MPA, NREMT-P

© 2011 American Heart Association
ISBN 978-1-61669-003-8
Printed in the United States of America
First American Heart Association Printing June 2011
10 9 8

Alexis Topjian, MD

Elise W. van der Jagt, MD, MPH

To find out about any updates or corrections to this text, visit **www.heart.org/cpr**, navigate to the page for this course, and click on "Updates."

Contents

Introduction

Welcome to the Family & Friends® CPR course. It's important that more people survive cardiac arrest. The greater the number of people who know CPR, the better someone's chances of surviving, so thanks for taking this course.

Heart attack, drowning, or other problems may cause someone's heart to stop pumping blood. This is called *cardiac arrest.* If you give a person CPR right away, he is more likely to survive. Most cardiac arrests happen at home with family members. You can help a loved one survive by doing CPR.

You will learn CPR through this manual and the video for the course. You'll have a chance to practice many times while the video guides you. When you aren't practicing with the video, you may watch the video or watch other students practice.

Use this manual in the following ways:

- Before the course: Read the manual.
- During the course: Use the manual to help you understand the information and skills.
- After the course: Review the manual. The more often you review, the better you'll remember.

This manual has the following modules:

Module 1

- CPR and AED for Adults: Hands-Only CPR
- Choking in Adults

Module 2

- CPR and AED for Children: Push and Give Breaths
- Choking in Children

Module 3

- CPR for Infants: Push and Give Breaths
- Choking in Infants

Thanks again for taking this course.

Module 1
CPR and AED for Adults:
Hands-Only CPR

What You Will Learn	By the end of this module you should know when to give CPR and be able to give CPR to an adult.
Definitions and Key Facts	CPR is the act of pushing hard and fast on the chest and giving breaths. It is given to someone whose heart has stopped pumping blood.
	In this module, you'll learn Hands-Only™ CPR. In Hands-Only CPR, you'll push hard and push fast, but you won't give breaths.
	In this module, when we refer to CPR, we mean Hands-Only CPR.
	For the purposes of this course, an adult is anyone who is going through or who has already gone through puberty.
	Someone who "responds" moves, speaks, blinks, or otherwise reacts to you when you tap him and ask if he's OK. Someone who doesn't "respond" does nothing when you tap him and ask if he's OK.
Topics in Hands-Only CPR	1. Give CPR: Push Hard and Push Fast 2. Use an AED 3. Assess and Phone 911 4. Put It All Together

Topic 1. Give CPR: Push Hard and Push Fast

Definitions and Key Facts

When you push on the chest, you pump blood to the brain and heart.

People often don't push hard enough because they're afraid of hurting the victim. An injury is unlikely, but it is better than death. It's better to push too hard than not hard enough. Occasionally, students worry they'll make an injury worse if they give an injured person CPR. They won't. If a person's heart has stopped, he won't survive. Your actions can only help.

Conventional CPR also involves giving breaths. But if someone needs CPR, you can do a lot of good by pushing hard and pushing fast.

Action: Give CPR

Follow these steps to push hard and push fast:

Step	Action
1	Make sure the person is lying on his back on a firm, flat surface.
2	Move clothes out of the way.
3	Put the heel of one hand on the lower half of the breastbone. Put the heel of your other hand on top of the first hand.
4	Push straight down **at least 2 inches** at a rate of **at least 100 pushes a minute.**
5	After each push, let the **chest come back up** to its normal position.

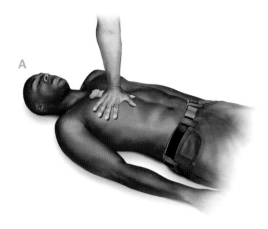

Figure 1. Pushing on the chest.
A, Put the heel of one hand on the lower half of the breastbone.
B, Put the other hand on top of the first hand.

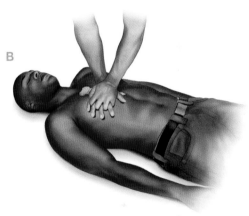

FYI

Pushing is important, and doing it right is tiring. The more tired you are, the less effective your pushes are. If someone else knows CPR, take turns pushing. Switch about every 2 minutes, moving quickly to keep the pause in pushing as short as possible. Remind each other to push down **at least 2 inches,** push at a rate of **at least 100 pushes a minute,** and let the **chest come back up** to its normal position after each push.

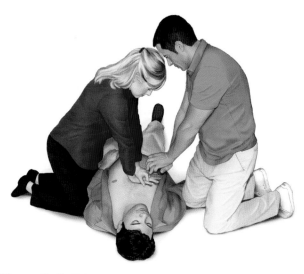

Figure 2. Switch rescuers.

Topic 2. Use an AED

Definitions and Key Facts

Sometimes a person's heart doesn't work right. An AED is a machine with a computer in it that can shock the heart and help it work properly again. If you start CPR right away and then use an AED within a few minutes, you will have the best chance of saving a life. AEDs are safe, accurate, and easy to use.

The AED is a machine that will figure out if the person needs a shock and will tell you to give one if it's needed. It will even tell you when to make sure that no one is touching the person. The pads used to shock the person have a diagram showing you where to place them. Follow the diagram.

The most common ways to turn on an AED are to push an "ON" button or lift the lid of the AED. Once you turn on the AED, it will tell you everything you need to do.

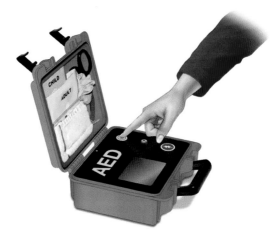

Figure 3. An automated external defibrillator (AED).

Actions

Use an AED if someone doesn't respond and isn't breathing or is only gasping. There are 2 steps for using an AED:

Step	Action
1	Turn the AED on.
2	Follow the prompts you see and hear.

Important

If you have access to an AED, use it as quickly as possible. If you can't find an AED quickly, then start CPR. Push hard and push fast.

Topic 3. Assess and Phone 911

Definitions and Key Facts

Now that you've learned how to give CPR, it's time to learn when to give CPR. The American Heart Association's adult Chain of Survival shows the most important actions you can take to deal with life-threatening emergencies.

The first link in the adult Chain is to recognize the emergency and phone for help. This is followed by early CPR with emphasis on pushing hard and fast, rapid AED use, effective advanced care, and coordinated care afterward.

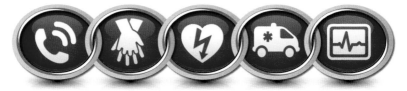

Figure 4. The adult Chain of Survival.

If you are not sure whether to give CPR, go ahead and give it. It's better to give CPR to someone who doesn't need it than to do nothing when someone does need CPR.

Action: Make Sure the Scene Is Safe

Before you assess the need for CPR, make sure the scene is safe. Look for anything nearby that might hurt you. You don't want to hurt yourself.

Action: Tap and Shout

Check if the person responds. Tap him and shout, "Are you OK?" If he doesn't move, speak, blink, or otherwise react, then he is not responding.

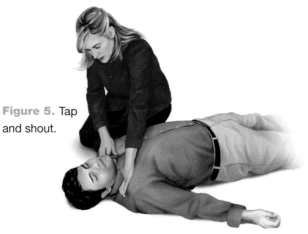

Figure 5. Tap and shout.

**Action:
Phone 911
and Get AED**

If the person doesn't respond, it's important to get help. You or someone else (yell for help if you need to) phone 911. Get an AED if one is available.

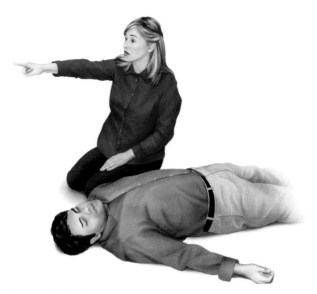

Figure 6. Get help.

**Action:
Check
Breathing**

If the person doesn't respond, check his breathing. Look from head to belly to see if the person is breathing. Do this for at least 5 seconds but no more than 10. If the person isn't breathing at all or if he is only "gasping," then he needs CPR.

A person who gasps usually looks like he is drawing air in very quickly. He may open his mouth and move the jaw, head, or neck. Gasps may appear forceful or weak, and some time may pass between gasps because they usually happen at a slow rate. The gasp may sound like a snort, snore, or groan. Gasping is not regular or normal breathing. It is a sign of cardiac arrest in someone who doesn't respond.

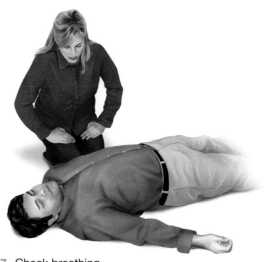

Figure 7. Check breathing.

FYI: Answering Dispatcher Questions

You need to stay on the phone until the 911 dispatcher (operator) tells you to hang up.

The dispatcher will ask you about the emergency. She may also tell you how to help the person until someone with more advanced training takes over.

Answering the dispatcher's questions will not delay the arrival of help. If you can, take the phone with you so that you are beside the person while you talk to the dispatcher.

Definitions and Key Facts

When doing CPR, push down **at least 2 inches** at a rate of **at least 100 pushes a minute.** After each push, let the **chest come back up** to its normal position.

Try not to interrupt pushing on the chest for more than a few seconds for any reason.

Action: Hands-Only CPR

The following table shows all the steps for Hands-Only CPR:

Step	Action
1	Make sure the scene is safe.
2	Tap and shout.
3	Yell for help. You or someone else **phone 911** and **get an AED.**
4	Check **breathing.**
5	If the person isn't responding and isn't breathing or is only gasping, then **give CPR.**
6	Keep pushing down **at least 2 inches** at a rate of **at least 100 pushes a minute,** allowing the **chest to come back up** to its normal position after each push, until the person starts to respond or someone with more advanced training takes over.

Hands-Only Review Sheet

Step	Action
1	**Make Sure the Scene Is Safe**
2	**Tap and Shout** ■ Check if the person responds. ■ If the person doesn't respond, then…
3	**Get Help** ■ Yell for help. ■ Have the person who comes phone 911 and get an AED. ■ If no one can help, phone 911 and get an AED.
4	**Check Breathing** ■ Make sure the person is on a firm, flat surface. ■ Check breathing. ■ If the person isn't breathing at all or if he is only gasping, then give CPR. **No response** + **No breathing or only gasping** = **GIVE CPR**
5	**Push Hard and Push Fast** ■ Pushes: – Move clothes out of the way. – Put the heel of one hand on the lower half of the breastbone. Put the heel of your other hand on top of the first hand. – Push straight down at least 2 inches at a rate of at least 100 pushes a minute. – After each push, let the chest come back up to its normal position. ■ AED: – Use it as soon as you have it. – Turn it on by lifting the lid or pressing the "ON" button. – Follow the prompts.
6	**Keep Going** ■ Keep pushing until the person starts to breathe or move or someone with more advanced training takes over.

Choking in Adults

What You Will Learn

By the end of this module you should be able to

- List the signs of choking
- Show how to help a choking adult

Definitions and Key Facts

Choking is when food or another object gets stuck in the airway or throat. The object stops air from getting to the lungs.

Some choking is mild and some is severe. If it's severe, act fast. Get the object out so the person can breathe.

Topics in Choking in Adults

1. Mild vs Severe Choking
2. How to Help a Choking Adult
3. How to Help a Choking Adult Who Stops Responding

Topic 1. Mild vs Severe Choking

Action

Use the following table to figure out if someone has mild or severe choking and what you should do:

If someone	The block in the airway is	And you should
• Can make sounds • Can cough loudly	Mild	• Stand by and let her cough • If you are worried about her breathing, phone 911

(continued)

If someone	The block in the airway is	And you should
• Cannot breathe or • Has a cough that has no sound or • Cannot talk or make a sound or • Makes the choking sign	Severe	• Act quickly • Follow the steps to help a choking adult

FYI: The Choking Sign

If someone is choking, he might use the choking sign (holding the neck with one or both hands).

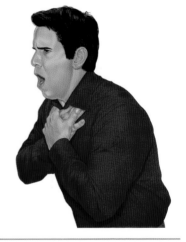

Figure 8. The choking sign: holding the neck with one or both hands.

Topic 2. How to Help a Choking Adult

Definitions and Key Facts

When someone has severe choking, give thrusts slightly above the belly button. These thrusts are sometimes called the *Heimlich maneuver.* Each thrust pushes air from the lungs like a cough. This can help remove an object blocking the airway.

Action: Help a Choking Adult

Follow these steps to help a choking adult:

Step	Action
1	If you think someone is choking, ask, "Are you choking?" If he nods yes, tell him you are going to help.
2	**Get behind him.** Wrap your arms around him so that your hands are in front.
3	**Make a fist** with one hand.
4	Put the thumb side of your fist slightly above the belly button and well below the breastbone.
5	**Grasp your fist with your other hand** and give quick upward thrusts into the belly.
6	**Give thrusts** until the object is forced out and he can breathe, cough, or talk, or until he stops responding.

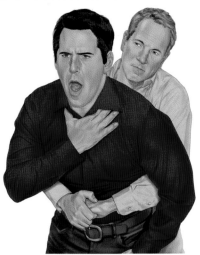

Figure 9. Helping someone who is choking.

Action:
Help a
Choking
Large Person
or Pregnant
Woman

If someone is choking and is in the late stages of pregnancy or is very large, give thrusts on the chest instead of thrusts on the belly.

Follow the same steps except for where you place your arms and hands. Put your arms under the person's armpits and your hands on the lower half of the breastbone. Pull straight back to give the chest thrusts.

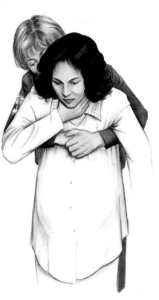

Figure 10. Chest thrusts on a choking large person or pregnant woman.

FYI

A person who has received thrusts should be seen by a healthcare provider.

Topic 3. How to Help a Choking Adult Who Stops Responding

Definitions
and Key
Facts

If you give someone thrusts but can't remove the object blocking the airway, the person will stop responding. Pushing on his chest may force the object out.

**Action:
Help a
Choking Adult
Who Stops
Responding**

If a choking adult stops responding, follow these steps:

Step	Action
1	Lower the choking adult to the ground, faceup.
2	Assess the need for CPR and phone 911.
3	Give CPR if it's needed.
4	Continue CPR until the person speaks, moves, or breathes, or someone with more advanced training takes over.

Module 2
CPR and AED for Children:
Push and Give Breaths

What You Will Learn

By the end of this module you should know when to give CPR and be able to give CPR to a child.

Definitions

CPR is the act of pushing hard and fast on the chest and giving breaths. CPR is given to someone whose heart has stopped pumping blood.

For the purposes of this course, a child is someone who is older than 1 year and has not yet reached puberty. If you are in doubt about whether someone is an adult or a child, treat the person as an adult.

A child who "responds" moves, speaks, blinks, or otherwise reacts to you when you tap him and ask if he's OK. A child who doesn't "respond" does nothing when you tap him and ask if he's OK.

Topics in CPR and AED for Children

1. Give CPR: Pushes and Breaths
2. Use an AED
3. Assess and Phone 911
4. Put It All Together

Topic 1. Give CPR: Pushes and Breaths

Push Hard and Push Fast

Definitions and Key Facts

Pushing hard and fast on the chest is the most important part of CPR. When you push on the chest, you pump blood to the brain and heart.

People often don't push hard enough because they're afraid of hurting the child. An injury is unlikely but it is better than death. It's better to push too hard than not hard enough. Occasionally, students worry they'll make an injury worse if they give an injured person CPR. They won't. If a person's heart has stopped, he won't survive. Your actions can only help.

Action: Push Hard and Push Fast

Follow these steps to push hard and push fast:

Step	Action
1	Make sure the child is lying on her back on a firm, flat surface.
2	Move clothes out of the way.
3	Put the heel of one hand on the lower half of the breastbone.
4	Push straight down **about 2 inches** at a rate of **at least 100 pushes a minute.**
5	After each push, let the **chest come back up** to its normal position.

FYI

Use one hand to push on a child's chest. If you can't push down about 2 inches with one hand, use two hands. One hand is not better than two or vice versa. Do what's necessary to push down about 2 inches.

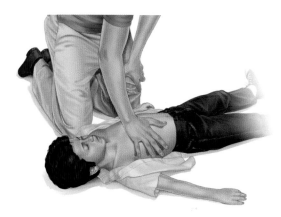

Figure 11. One-handed compressions.

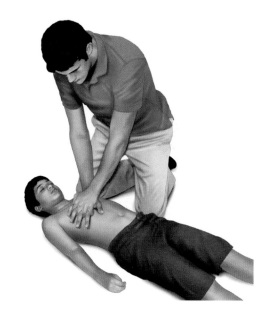

Figure 12. Two-handed compressions.

Pushing is important, and doing it right is tiring. The more tired you are, the less effective your pushes are. If someone else knows CPR, take turns. Switch rescuers about every 2 minutes, moving quickly so that the pause in pushing is as short as possible. Remind each other to push down **about 2 inches,** to push at a rate of **at least 100 pushes a minute,** and to let the **chest come back up** to its normal position after each push.

Give Breaths

Definitions and Key Facts

Children often have healthy hearts. Usually a child's heart stops because she can't breathe or is having trouble breathing. As a result, it's very important to give breaths as well as chest pushes to a child.

Your breaths need to make the child's chest rise. When the chest rises, you know the child has gotten enough air. Pushing on the chest is the most important part of CPR. If you are also able to give breaths, you will help the child even more.

Action: Open the Airway

Before giving breaths, open the airway. Follow these steps to open the airway:

Step	Action
1	Put one hand on the forehead and the fingers of your other hand on the bony part of the child's chin.
2	Tilt the head back and lift the chin.

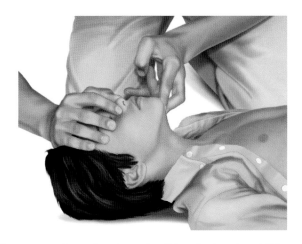

Figure 13. Open the airway by tilting the head and lifting the chin.

Important   Avoid pressing on the soft part of the neck or under the chin.

Action: Give Breaths   Follow these steps to give breaths to a child:

Step	Action
1	While holding the child's airway open, take a normal breath.
2	Pinch the nose shut. Cover the child's mouth with your mouth.
3	**Give 2 breaths** (blow for 1 second each). Watch for the **chest to rise** as you give each breath.

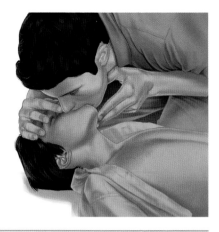

Figure 14. Cover the child's mouth with your mouth.

Important

If you give a child a breath and the chest doesn't rise, reopen the airway by allowing the head to go back to the normal position. Then open the airway again by tilting the head and lifting the chin. Then give another breath. Make sure the chest rises.

Don't interrupt pushes for more than 10 seconds to give breaths. If the chest doesn't rise within 10 seconds, begin pushing hard and pushing fast on the chest again.

Topic 2. Use an AED

Definitions and Key Facts

Sometimes a person's heart doesn't work right. An AED is a machine with a computer in it that can shock the heart and help it work properly again. If you start CPR right away and use an AED within a few minutes, you will have the best chance of saving a life. AEDs are safe, accurate, and easy to use.

The AED will figure out if the child needs a shock and will tell you to give one if it's needed. It will even tell you when to make sure that no one is touching the child. Some AEDs may have pads for a child, a child key, or a child switch. The pads used to shock the child have a diagram showing you where to place them. Follow the diagram.

The most common ways to turn on an AED are to push an "ON" button or lift the lid of the AED. Once you turn on the AED, it will tell you everything you need to do.

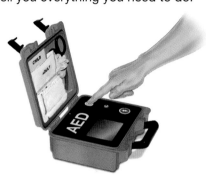

Figure 15.
An automated external defibrillator (AED).

Action

Use an AED on any child who needs CPR. There are 4 simple steps for using an AED on a child:

Step	Action
1	Turn the AED on.
2	Look for child pads or for a child key or switch.
3	Use the child pads or turn the child key or switch.
4	Follow the prompts you see and hear.

Important

If there are no child pads or if there isn't a child key or switch, use the adult pads. When you put the pads on the chest, make sure they don't touch each other.

If you have access to an AED, use it as quickly as possible. If you can't find an AED quickly, don't wait. Start CPR.

Definitions and Key Facts

Now that you've learned how to give CPR, it's time to learn when to give CPR. If a child doesn't respond and if that child isn't breathing or is only gasping, then you need to give CPR.

If you are not sure whether or not to give CPR, go ahead and give it. It's better to give CPR to someone who doesn't need it than to do nothing when someone does need CPR.

Action: Make Sure the Scene Is Safe

Before you give CPR, make sure the scene is safe. Look for anything nearby that might hurt you. You don't want to hurt yourself.

Action: Tap and Shout

Check if the child responds. Tap him and shout, "Are you OK?" If he doesn't move, speak, blink, talk, or otherwise react, then he is not responding.

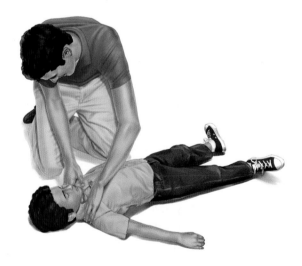

Figure 16. Tap and shout.

**Action:
Yell for Help**

Yell for help. If someone comes, have that person phone 911 and get an AED. Whether or not someone comes, check the child's breathing next.

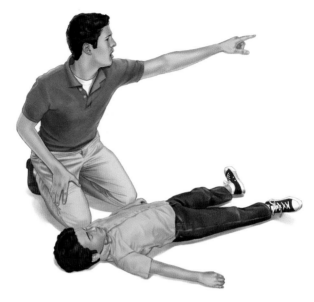

Figure 17. Get help.

**Action:
Check
Breathing**

If the child doesn't respond, check his breathing. Look from head to belly to see if the child is breathing. Do this for at least 5 seconds but no more than 10. If the child isn't breathing at all or if he is only "gasping," then he needs CPR.

A person who gasps usually looks like he is drawing air in very quickly. He may open his mouth and move the jaw, head, or neck. Gasps may appear forceful or weak, and some time may pass between gasps because they usually happen at a slow rate. The gasp may sound like a snort, snore, or groan. Gasping is not regular or normal breathing. It is a sign of cardiac arrest in someone who doesn't respond.

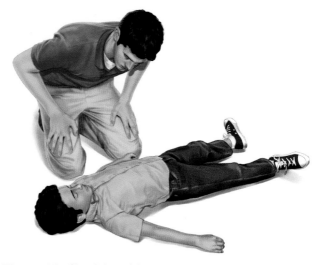

Figure 18. Check breathing.

Topic 4. Put It All Together

Definitions and Key Facts

Because children's hearts are often healthy and breathing trouble is often the cause of the child's heart problem, it's important to get air to the child as fast as possible. For this reason, you should give 5 sets of CPR before phoning for help or getting an AED.

Pushing is very important and is the core of CPR. Try not to interrupt pushing on the chest for more than a few seconds, even when you give breaths.

Action: Give 5 Sets of CPR

When doing CPR, you **give sets of 30 pushes and 2 breaths.** Push **about 2 inches** at a rate of **at least 100 pushes a minute.** After each push, let the **chest come back up** to its normal position.

If the child doesn't respond and isn't breathing or is only gasping, then give him 5 sets of CPR (1 set = 30 pushes and 2 breaths).

Action: Phone and Get an AED	After 5 sets of CPR, phone 911 and get an AED if no one has done this yet. As soon as you have the AED, use it.

Action: Keep Going	After phoning 911, keep giving sets of 30 pushes and 2 breaths until the child begins to respond or someone with more advanced training arrives and takes over.

FYI: Answering Dispatcher Questions	You need to stay on the phone until the 911 dispatcher (operator) tells you to hang up.

The dispatcher will ask you about the emergency. She may also tell you how to help the child until someone with more advanced training takes over.

Answering the dispatcher's questions will not delay the arrival of help. If you can, take the phone with you so that you are beside the child while you talk to the dispatcher. |

Action: Child CPR

No response + No breathing or only gasping = GIVE CPR

The following table shows the steps for child CPR:

Step	Action
1	Make sure the scene is safe.
2	Tap and shout.
3	Yell for help.
4	Check breathing.
5	If the child isn't responding and either isn't breathing or is only gasping, **give 5 sets of 30 pushes and 2 breaths, and then phone 911 and get an AED.**

(continued)

(continued)

Step	Action
6	Keep giving **sets of pushes and breaths** until the child starts to speak, breathe, or move, or someone with more advanced training takes over.

Important

If another person is with you when you give CPR— or if you can yell for help and get someone to come help you—then send the other person or people to phone 911 while you start pushing hard and fast and giving breaths. **You push and give breaths; they phone and get the AED.**

Child Review Sheet

Step	Action
1	**Make Sure the Scene Is Safe**
2	**Tap and Shout** ■ Check if the child responds. ■ If the child doesn't respond, then…
3	**Yell for Help** ■ See if there's someone who can help you. ■ Have that person phone 911 and get an AED.
4	**Check Breathing** ■ Make sure the child is on a firm, flat surface. ■ See if the child is not breathing or is only gasping. **No response** + **No breathing or only gasping** = **GIVE CPR**

5	**Give CPR**
	■ Give 5 sets of 30 pushes and 2 breaths, and then phone 911 and get an AED (if no one has done this yet).
	■ Push hard and fast:
	  – Move clothes out of the way.
	  – Put the heel of one hand on the lower half of the breastbone.
	  – Push straight down about 2 inches at a rate of at least 100 pushes a minute.
	  – After each push, let the chest come back up to its normal position.
	  – Push on the chest 30 times.
	■ Give breaths:
	  – After 30 pushes, open the airway with a head tilt–chin lift.
	  – After the airway is open, take a normal breath.
	  – Pinch the nose shut. Cover the child's mouth with your mouth.
	  – Give 2 breaths (blow for 1 second each). Watch for the chest to rise as you give each breath.
	■ AED:
	  – Use it as soon as you have it.
	  – Turn it on by pressing the "ON" button or lifting the lid.
	  – Use the child pads or turn the child key or switch. (Use the adult pads if there are no child pads.)
	  – Follow the prompts.

6	**Keep Going** ■ Keep giving sets of pushes and breaths until the child starts to speak, breathe, or move, or someone with more advanced training takes over.

Choking in Children

What You Will Learn

By the end of this module you should be able to

- List the signs of choking
- Show how to help a choking child

Definitions and Key Facts

Choking is when food or another object gets stuck in the airway or throat. The object stops air from getting to the lungs.

Some choking is mild and some is severe. If it's severe, act fast. Get the object out so the child can breathe.

Topics in Choking in Children

1. Mild vs Severe Choking
2. How to Help a Choking Child
3. How to Help a Choking Child Who Stops Responding

Topic 1. Mild vs Severe Choking

Action

Use the following table to figure out if a child has mild or severe choking and what you should do.

If the child	The block in the airway is	And you should
• Can make sounds • Can cough loudly	Mild	• Stand by and let her cough • If you are worried about the child's breathing, phone 911

(continued)

(continued)

If the child	The block in the airway is	And you should
• Cannot breathe or • Has a cough that has no sound or • Cannot talk or make a sound or • Makes the choking sign	Severe	• Act quickly • Follow the steps to help a choking child

FYI: The Choking Sign

If a child is choking, she might use the choking sign (holding the neck with one or both hands).

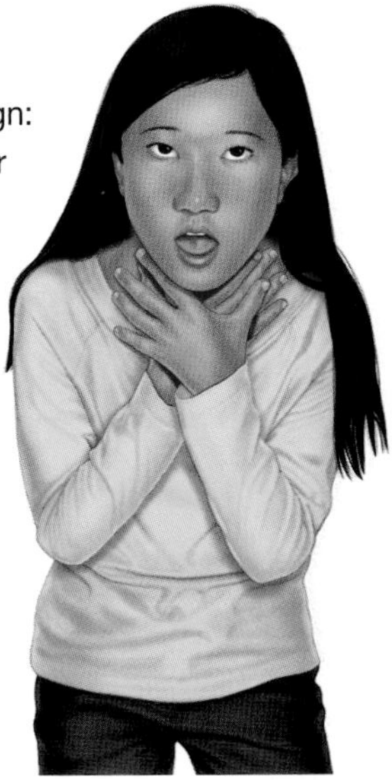

Figure 19. The choking sign: holding the neck with one or both hands.

Topic 2. How to Help a Choking Child

Definitions and Key Facts

When a child has severe choking, give thrusts slightly above the belly button. These thrusts are sometimes called the *Heimlich maneuver.* Each thrust pushes air from the lungs like a cough. This can help remove an object blocking the airway.

Action: Help a Choking Child

Follow these steps to help a choking child:

Step	Action
1	If you think the child is choking, ask, "Are you choking?" If she nods yes, tell her you are going to help.
2	**Get behind her.** Wrap your arms around her so that your hands are in front.
3	**Make a fist** with one hand.
4	Put the thumb side of your fist slightly above the belly button and well below the breastbone.
5	**Grasp your fist with your other hand** and give quick upward thrusts into the belly.
6	**Give thrusts** until the object is forced out and she can breathe, cough, or talk, or until she stops responding.

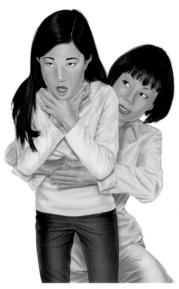

Figure 20. Helping a choking child.

Action: Help a Choking Large Child

If the choking child is very large, give thrusts on the chest instead of thrusts on the belly.

Follow the same steps except for where you place your arms and hands. Put your arms under the child's armpits and your hands on the lower half of the breastbone. Pull straight back to give the chest thrusts.

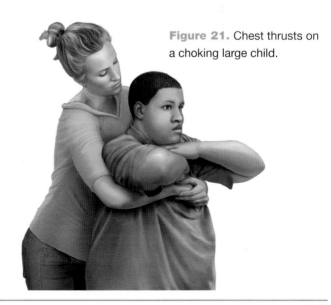

Figure 21. Chest thrusts on a choking large child.

FYI   A child who has been given thrusts should see a healthcare provider.

Topic 3. How to Help a Choking Child Who Stops Responding

Definitions and Key Facts

If you give a child thrusts but can't remove the object blocking the airway, the child will stop responding. Pushing on his chest may force the object out.

Action: Help a Choking Child Who Stops Responding

If the child stops responding, follow these steps:

Step	Action
1	Lower the child to a firm, flat surface.
2	Tap and shout.
3	**Yell for help.**
4	**Check breathing.**
5	**Push on the chest 30 times.**
6	After 30 pushes, open the airway. **If you see an object in the child's mouth, take it out.**
7	**Give 2 breaths.**
8	**Repeat** giving **sets of 30 pushes and 2 breaths,** checking the mouth for objects after each set of pushes.
9	**After 5 sets of 30 pushes and 2 breaths, phone** 911 and get an AED (if no one has done this).
10	**Give sets of 30 pushes and 2 breaths,** checking the mouth for objects after each set of pushes, until the child starts to respond or someone with more advanced training takes over.

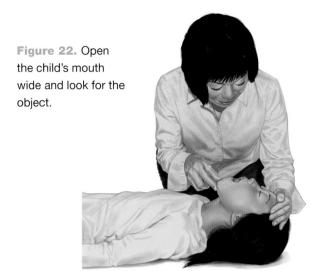

Figure 22. Open the child's mouth wide and look for the object.

Module 3
CPR for Infants:
Push and Give Breaths

What You Will Learn

By the end of this module you should know when to give CPR and be able to give CPR to an infant.

Definitions and Key Facts

CPR is the act of pushing hard and fast on the chest and giving breaths. CPR is given to someone whose heart has stopped pumping blood.

For the purposes of this course, an infant is younger than 1 year.

An infant who "responds" moves, makes sounds, blinks, or otherwise reacts to you when you tap him and shout something, such as his name. An infant who doesn't "respond" does nothing when you tap him and shout.

Topics in CPR for Infants

1. Give CPR: Pushes and Breaths
2. Assess and Phone 911
3. Put It All Together

Topic 1. Give CPR:
Pushes and Breaths

Push Hard and Push Fast

Definitions and Key Facts

Pushing hard and fast on the chest is the most important part of CPR. When you push on the chest, you pump blood to the brain and heart.

People often don't push hard enough because they're afraid of hurting the infant. An injury is unlikely, but it is better than death. It's better to push too hard than not hard enough. Occasionally, students worry they'll make an injury worse if they give an injured infant CPR. They won't. If an infant's heart has stopped, he won't survive. Your actions can only help.

If possible, place the infant on a firm, flat surface above the ground, such as a table. This makes it easier to give CPR.

Action: Push Hard and Push Fast

Follow these steps to push hard and push fast:

Step	Action
1	Make sure the infant is lying on her back on a firm, flat surface above the ground.
2	Move clothes out of the way.
3	Put 2 fingers of one hand on the breastbone just below the nipple line.
4	Press the infant's chest straight down **about 1½ inches** at a rate of **at least 100 pushes a minute.**
5	After each push, let the **chest come back up** to its normal position.

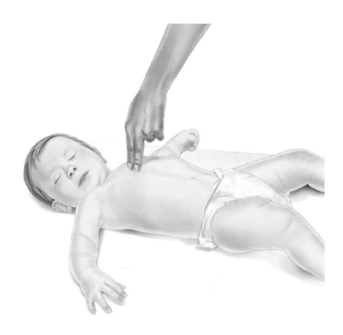

Figure 23. Put 2 fingers just below the nipple line. Avoid the tip of breastbone.

FYI

Pushing is important, and doing it right is tiring. The more tired you are, the less effective your pushes are. If someone else knows CPR, take turns. Switch rescuers about every 2 minutes, moving quickly so that the pause in pushing is as short as possible. Remind each other to push down **about 1½ inches,** to push at a rate of **at least 100 pushes a minute,** and to let the **chest come back up** to its normal position after each push.

Give Breaths

Definitions and Key Facts

Infants often have healthy hearts. Usually an infant's heart stops because she can't breathe or is having trouble breathing. As a result, it's very important to give breaths as well as chest pushes to an infant.

Your breaths need to make the infant's chest rise. When the chest rises, you know the infant has gotten enough air. Pushing on the chest is the most important part of CPR. If you are also able to give breaths, you will help the infant even more.

Action: Open the Airway

Before giving breaths, open the airway. Follow these steps to open the airway:

Step	Action
1	Put one hand on the forehead and the fingers of your other hand on the bony part of the infant's chin.
2	Tilt the head back and lift the chin.

Important

When tilting an infant's head, do not push it back too far because this may block the infant's airway. Avoid pressing the soft part of the neck or under the chin.

Action: Give Breaths

Follow these steps to give breaths to an infant:

Step	Action
1	While holding the infant's airway open, take a normal breath.
2	Cover the infant's mouth and nose with your mouth.
3	**Give 2 breaths** (blow for 1 second each). Watch for the **chest to rise** as you give each breath.

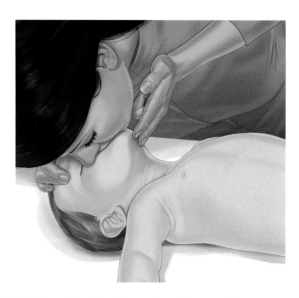

Figure 24. Cover the infant's mouth and nose with your mouth.

FYI: Tips for Giving Breaths

If your mouth is too small to cover the infant's mouth and nose, put your mouth over the infant's nose and give breaths through the infant's nose. (You may need to hold the infant's mouth closed to stop air from coming out through the mouth.)

Important

If you give an infant a breath and the chest doesn't rise, reopen the airway by allowing the head to go back to the normal position. Then open the airway again by tilting the head and lifting the chin. Then give another breath. Make sure the chest rises.

Don't interrupt pushes for more than 10 seconds to give breaths. If the chest doesn't rise within 10 seconds, begin pushing hard and pushing fast on the chest again.

Definitions and Key Facts	Now that you've learned how to give CPR, it's time to learn when to give CPR. If an infant doesn't respond and if that infant isn't breathing or is only gasping, then you need to give CPR.
	If you are not sure whether or not to give CPR, go ahead and give it. It's better to give CPR to someone who doesn't need it than to do nothing when someone does need CPR.
Action: Make Sure the Scene Is Safe	Before you give CPR, make sure the scene is safe. Look for anything nearby that might hurt you. You don't want to hurt yourself.
Action: Tap and Shout	Check if the infant responds. Tap his foot and shout his name. If he doesn't move, make sounds, blink, or otherwise react, then he is not responding.

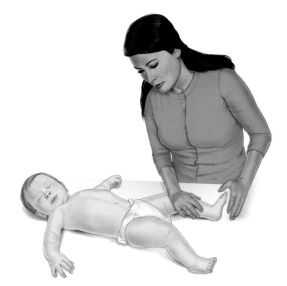

Figure 25. Tap and shout.

Action:
Yell for Help

Yell for help. If someone comes, have that person phone 911. Whether or not someone comes, check the child's breathing next.

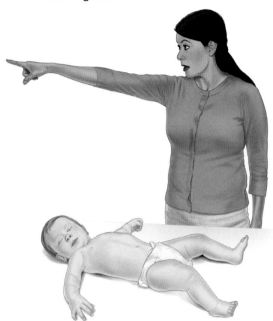

Figure 26. Get help.

Action:
Check
Breathing

If the infant doesn't respond, check his breathing. Look from head to belly to see if the infant is breathing. Do this for at least 5 seconds but no more than 10. If the infant isn't breathing at all or if he is only "gasping," then he needs CPR.

A person who gasps usually looks like he is drawing air in very quickly. He may open his mouth and move the jaw, head, or neck. Gasps may appear forceful or weak, and some time may pass between gasps because they usually happen at a slow rate. The gasp may sound like a snort, snore, or groan. Gasping is not regular or normal breathing. It is a sign of cardiac arrest in someone who doesn't respond.

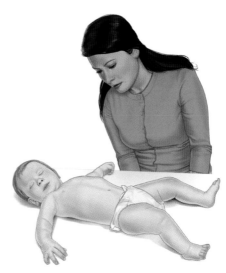

Figure 27. Check breathing.

Topic 3. Put It All Together

Definitions and Key Facts

Because infants' hearts are often healthy and because breathing trouble is often the cause of the infant's heart problem, it's important to get air to the infant as fast as possible. For this reason, you should give 5 sets of CPR before phoning for help.

Pushing is very important and is the core of CPR. Try not to interrupt pushing on the chest for more than a few seconds, even when you give breaths.

**Action:
Give 5 Sets
of CPR**

When doing CPR, you **give sets of 30 pushes and 2 breaths.** Push down **about 1½ inches** at a rate of **at least 100 pushes a minute.** After each push, let the **chest come back up** to its normal position.

If the infant is not injured and you are alone, after 5 sets of 30 pushes and 2 breaths, you may carry the infant with you to phone 911.

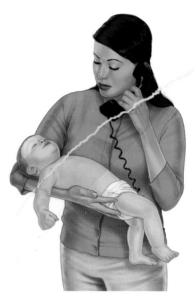

Figure 28. Phone 911.

**Action:
Phone 911**

After 5 sets of CPR, phone 911 if no one has done this yet. Take the infant with you to the phone if possible.

**Action:
Keep Going**

After phoning, keep giving sets of 30 pushes and 2 breaths until the infant begins to respond or someone with more advanced training arrives and takes over.

You need to stay on the phone until the 911 dispatcher (operator) tells you to hang up.

The dispatcher will ask you about the emergency. She may also tell you how to help the infant until someone with more advanced training takes over.

Answering the dispatcher's questions will not delay the arrival of help. If you can, take the infant with you to the phone while you talk to the dispatcher.

**Action:
Infant CPR**

| No response | + | No breathing
or
only gasping | = | GIVE CPR |

The following table shows the steps for infant CPR:

Step	Action
1	Make sure the scene is safe.
2	Tap and shout.
3	Yell for help.
4	Check breathing.
5	If the infant isn't responding and either isn't breathing or is only gasping, **give 5 sets of 30 pushes and 2 breaths, and then phone 911.**
6	Keep giving **sets of pushes and breaths** until the infant starts to breathe or move or someone with more advanced training takes over.

Important

If another person is with you when you give CPR— or if you can yell for help and get someone to come help you—then send the other person or people to phone 911 while you start pushing hard and fast and giving breaths. **You push and give breaths; they phone.**

Infant Review Sheet

Step	Action
1	**Make Sure the Scene Is Safe**
2	**Tap and Shout** ■ Check if the infant responds. ■ If the infant doesn't respond, then…
3	**Yell for Help** ■ See if there's someone who can help you. ■ Have that person phone 911.
4	**Check Breathing** ■ Make sure the infant is on a firm, flat surface above the ground. ■ See if the infant isn't breathing at all or is only gasping. **No response** + **No breathing or only gasping** = **GIVE CPR**
5	**Give CPR** ■ Give 5 sets of 30 pushes and 2 breaths, and then phone 911 (if no one has phoned yet). ■ Pushes: – Move clothes out of the way. – Place 2 fingers just below the nipple line. – Push straight down about 1½ inches at a rate of at least 100 pushes a minute. – After each push, let the chest come back up to its normal position. – Push on the chest 30 times. ■ Give breaths: – After 30 pushes, open the airway with a head tilt–chin lift. – After the airway is open, take a normal breath. – Cover the infant's mouth and nose with your mouth. – Give 2 breaths (blow for 1 second each). Watch for the chest to rise as you give each breath.
6	**Keep Going** ■ Keep giving sets of pushes and breaths until the infant starts to breathe or move or someone with more advanced training takes over.

Choking in Infants

What You Will Learn	By the end of this module you should be able to ■ List the signs of choking ■ Show how to help a choking infant
Definitions and Key Facts	Choking is when food or another object gets stuck in the airway or throat. The object stops air from getting to the lungs. Some choking is mild and some is severe. If it's severe, act fast. Get the object out so the infant can breathe.
Topics in Choking in Infants	1. Mild vs Severe Choking 2. How to Help a Choking Infant 3. How to Help a Choking Infant Who Stops Responding

Topic 1. Mild vs Severe Choking

Action	Use the following table to figure out if an infant has mild or severe choking and what you should do.

If the infant	The block in the airway is	And you should
• Can make sounds • Can cough loudly	Mild	• Stand by and let her cough • If you are worried about the infant's breathing, phone 911

(continued)

50

(continued)

If the infant	The block in the airway is	And you should
• Cannot breathe or • Has a cough that has no sound or • Cannot make a sound	Severe	• Act quickly • Follow the steps to help a choking infant

Topic 2. How to Help a Choking Infant

Definitions and Key Facts

When an infant has severe choking, use back slaps and chest thrusts to help remove the object blocking the airway.

Action: Help a Choking Infant

Follow these steps to help a choking infant:

Step	Action
1	Hold the infant facedown on your forearm. Support the infant's head and jaw with your hand.
2	Give up to **5 back slaps** with the heel of your other hand between the infant's shoulder blades.
3	If the object does not come out after 5 back slaps, turn the infant onto his back, supporting the head.
4	Give up to **5 chest thrusts** using 2 fingers of your other hand to push on the chest in the same place you push during CPR.
5	**Repeat** giving 5 back slaps and 5 chest thrusts until the infant can breathe, cough, or cry, or until he stops responding.

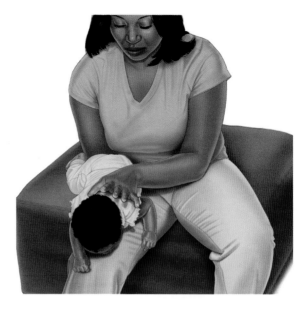

Figure 29. Give up to 5 back slaps.

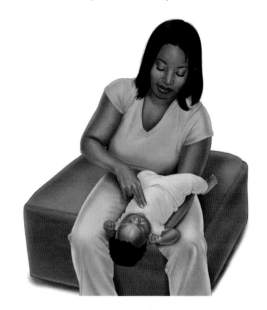

Figure 30. Give up to 5 chest thrusts.

FYI

An infant who has been given back slaps and chest thrusts should be seen by a healthcare provider.

Topic 3. How to Help a Choking Infant Who Stops Responding

Definitions and Key Facts

If you give an infant back slaps and chest thrusts and can't remove the object blocking the airway, the infant will stop responding. Pushing on his chest may force the object out.

Action: Help a Choking Infant Who Stops Responding

If the infant stops responding, follow these steps:

Step	Action
1	Place the infant faceup on a firm, flat surface above the ground, such as a table.
2	Tap and shout.
3	**Yell for help.**
4	**Check breathing.**
5	**Push on the chest 30 times.**
6	After 30 pushes, open the airway. **If you see an object in the mouth, take it out.**
7	**Give 2 breaths.**
8	**Repeat** giving **sets of 30 pushes and 2 breaths,** checking the mouth for objects after each set of pushes.
9	**After 5 sets of 30 pushes and 2 breaths, phone 911.**
10	**Give sets of 30 pushes and 2 breaths,** checking the mouth for objects after each set of pushes, until the infant starts to respond or someone with more advanced training arrives and takes over.

Important   Giving thrusts to an infant's belly could cause serious harm. Only give back slaps and chest thrusts to an infant.

If another person is with you when the infant stops responding—or if you can yell for help and get someone to come help you—then send the other person or people to phone 911 while you start pushing hard and fast and giving breaths. **You push and give breaths; they phone.**

Conclusion

Congratulations! Thanks for taking time to attend this course.

Few people do CPR perfectly from start to finish. Of course, in an ideal world, everyone would do it perfectly. But even imperfect CPR can help save a life. When someone needs CPR, pushing hard and pushing fast never hurts and often helps. So push on the chest. And remember to phone 911. The dispatcher can remind you what to do.

Contact the American Heart Association if you want more information on CPR, AEDs, or first aid. Visit **www.heart.org/cpr** or call 877-AHA-4CPR (877-242-4277) to find a class near you.

It's important to save as many lives as possible through CPR. Thank you for joining us in this mission.